Caring for Elderly Patients

Help and Guidance from a Sympathetic Doctor Who Has Lived It

By: Jack Rosenberg, M.D.

Caregivers Advisors

1003 Willow Creek Road
Prescott, AZ 86301
www.CaregiversAdvisors.org

Copyright © 2013 by Jack Rosenberg, M.D.
All rights reserved. No part of this book may be copied, transmitted or stored in a database without permission.

DISCLAIMER

This book is not intended as medical advice. It is also not intended to prevent, diagnose, treat or cure disease. Instead the book is intended only to share the unofficial research and opinion of the author. The information is provided for educational purposes only, not as treatment instructions for any disease or ailment. Much of the book is a statement of opinion in areas where the facts are controversial or do not exist. The information in this book should not be considered any more valid than any other type of informal opinion.

The information was not written to replace the advice or care of a qualified health care professional. Be sure to check with your own qualified health care provider before beginning any protocols or procedures discussed in this book, or before stopping or altering any diet, lifestyle, or other therapies previously recommended to you by your health care provider.

The treatments described in this book may have side effects and carry other known and unknown risks and health hazards. The statements in this book have not been evaluated by the United States FDA. Use of the information in this book is at your own risk.

This book is dedicated to Mrs. JoAnne Lerner, our loving mother, who currently lives with us, and suffers from severe dementia. She is loving, caring and never stops amazing us.

A Message to All Struggling Caregivers

Sometimes life turns around and the person who has taken care of you all your life starts to need care themselves. If your loved one is also dealing with degenerative diseases like Alzheimer's or dementia it's a big task not only for you but for the whole family as well.

I am Dr. Jack Rosenberg. My wife's mother is suffering from severe dementia and we have gone down the same road that you are walking on right now; facing the same heartbreaking decisions that you face. It is my purpose to empower you to make good decisions for your loved one's health using the knowledge and experience I've obtained as a medical doctor for the past 20+ years.

It was months of frustration for me to learn the ins and outs of all the documentation, legal forms and information that I needed to compile in order to get the treatment necessary for my mother-in-law. Finally, to alleviate the stress, I organized the whole mess into my Go-to-Packet. This is an essential guide I use to help my own mother-in-law and it will help alleviate the stress of caregiving for you too.

Normally sold for $9.95, I've made my Go-to-Packet available at http://caregiversadvisors.org/go-to for you to download at no charge.

I hope that by downloading the Go-to-Packet and reading this book, you'll change your perspective and get organized to make caring for your loved ones a little easier. For all your inquiries on caregiving, feel free to send me an email.

All the best,
Dr. Jack Rosenberg
drrosenberg@caregiversadvisors.org

Table of Contents

Chapter 1- My Wife's Story 7

Chapter 2- Diagnosing and Understanding Alzheimer's Disease 10

Chapter 3- Taking Legal Responsibility for an Alzheimer's or Dementia Patient 12

Chapter 4- Choosing Nursing Care for Your Loved One with Alzheimer's 15

Chapter 5- Is Home Health Care the Best Decision for My Loved One? 18

Chapter 6- Helping Those Caring for Parents with Alzheimer's and Dementia 21

Chapter 7- Working with Doctors and Memory Loss Patients 23

Chapter 8- Getting the Needed Support 26

Chapter 9- Communication with an Alzheimer's Patient 28

Chapter 10- Helping Kids Understand Alzheimer's and Dementia . 32

Chapter 11- Elderly Exercises 35

Chapter 12- Tips for Caregivers of Alzheimer's Patients 38

Chapter 13- When Caring for an Alzheimer's Patient 42

Chapter 14- Understanding Memory Loss 45

Chapter 15- Elderly Health Concerns 48

Recommended Reading 51

About The Author 55

Chapter 1 - My Wife's Story

My name is Jennifer, and I'm a 49 year old mom of a busy 17 year old son and a 15 year old daughter, and a wife of 22 years of a medical doctor. And, of course, I must mention my two golden retrievers.

Chances are when my parents paid for me to go to college and get a Bachelor in Science degree as an occupational therapist 30 years ago; they didn't think my education would benefit them in any way. Fortunately, I spent my entire career as a therapist treating patients in an in-patient rehab unit. That experience gave me the knowledge and expertise to be able to help my parents navigate through their physical and mental disabilities later in life.

About ten years ago my husband and I decided to help my parents move across the country to live closer to us so we could help advocate for my father with his health care. Unfortunately, he passed away four years ago after the ramifications of a horrible disease of diabetes. He ended up with several disabilities; for example, he was a bilateral amputee of his lower extremities, he lost his vision, he lost his hearing, he was on dialysis three times a week, he had multiple surgeries, which of course has always setbacks for a patient of that diagnosis. It was a blessing that we were able to help him with his health care. Being in the healthcare field, we were able to provide him the best possible life he could have being as handicapped as he was.

Since my father had passed away, the last six years of my mother's life has been interesting. Little did we know that she was displaying signs of dementia. Little by little, unfortunately, we were so focused on my father's disabilities that we ignored the signs. Had we recognized that she was showing signs of dementia, perhaps we could've gotten her on medications to slow down the process. As time went by, it became apparent to us that she could no longer live alone. She began getting lost around town, going to work at the wrong times on the wrong days and, worst off, getting in multiple car accidents and not remembering them.

After a year of trying to get her out of her independent living environment to keep her safer, we looked into a variety of different supervised living situations. We explored every possible avenue there is. When it came down to it, we came to a conclusion that the best thing for our family would be to move her in with us.

Fortunately for us, my mother is a very pleasant, happy-go-lucky dementia patient. So, the burden of taking care of her is more on setting her up with activities and keeping her life as fulfilled as possible. Initially, moving her in with us was a burden. There was a lot of stress not only for myself and my wife, but also the family. It's not easy to bring another family member into your household when you're already set in your ways and busy.

It has now been a little more than a year since she has lived with us, and things seem to be going pretty smoothly. We figured out ways to utilize services in the community. For example, we have an adult activity center that sends a bus to drive her both ways. She thinks that she's going to work on those three days when she goes there and she feels very useful and proud of the work that she thinks she does there. It gives her a sense of fulfillment and it gives us a break that she leaves and goes to her activity center.

After all the work that we did to plug my mom in, we decided as a family that we should share our knowledge as health care professionals. We have learned a lot in the last couple of years exploring all the different supervised living places in our town. Hopefully, utilizing our expertise in caring for the aging Alzheimer's dementia patient, this information can help in making it a little bit easier for you.

CHAPTER 2- DIAGNOSING AND UNDERSTANDING ALZHEIMER'S DISEASE

Alzheimer's disease is known as the most common form of dementia. Dementia is a term used to describe the loss of a person's memory and other abilities that affect their daily life.

People that care for others with Alzheimer's, can find it very challenging at times to deal with. Many family members care for loved ones with the disease, or place them in a type of facility where they are able to receive the appropriate care they need.

Alzheimer's diagnosis is sometimes fairly easy for physicians to provide to the patient and their family, as the signs of this illness is very familiar to them. When signs of memory loss become obvious in people, it is best to see a physician as soon as possible, because many people find it to be harder to realize there is a true issue going on with them. People often care for their loved ones at home, and most often, the loved one is a parent. When a parent is diagnosed with dementia, it may be harder for the one caring for them to understand and cope with everything about the illness.

Many people are already struggling with coping with the aging process, and being diagnosed with Alzheimer's and dementia, only adds to the stress that they already have. It is already harder for the older person to lose their independence, but they can experience many other feelings such as confusion, anger, depression, and feelings of loneliness. Responses from being diagnosed with the disease are different, and many respond in a very negative way to while others learn to accept the fact of being diagnosed with the disease.

There are many family members along with the patient that have a very difficult time accepting it, and coping with it. Alzheimer's diagnosis can cause a person's whole lifestyle to change, and it can have an effect on other family members as well. People that are diagnosed with the disease do have options to choose from as far as living conditions.

Although Alzheimer's is an irreversible illness, patients and their families can still live a whole, enjoyable life at home. Depending on the severity of the illness, many people may want to place their loved ones in some type of a facility, or continue to care for them at home.

Family members caring for a loved one that has been diagnosed with Alzheimer's and dementia may not be aware that help is always available when they need assistance.

The Alzheimer's Association is available for any information caregivers may need, or questions that patients and caregivers may have. Patients and family need to realize that they are never alone in these types of situations, as there are many people across America, that suffer from this type of illness. Being there for the patient and loved ones, is one of the more important things in these types of situations. Knowing that they have someone who cares is the best thing for the patient. In time, some patients learn to adapt to their new lifestyle changes, while many others may never accept it.

Chapter 3 - Taking Legal Responsibility for an Alzheimer's or Dementia Patient

Your parent or loved ones' diagnosis with Alzheimer's or dementia could have come as a shock to you, even if you already knew deep down that something wasn't right with them anymore. You will need an emotional adjustment period. While it is important that you give yourself the time to process these developments, time is of the essence when it comes to your loved ones' finances.

Taking legal responsibility for parents, or other loved ones, can be a time consuming process. It needs to be begun as soon as the realization is made that within a very short time they will no longer be able to handle their own finances. There will be many decisions to be made and legal documents to process. This is optimally done while the patient is still in a relatively sound mind.

Some areas to consider before beginning this process are:

1. Be respectful. The first consideration at hand is your parent or loved one's feelings. They have spent a lifetime being in control of their own lives, and it will be difficult for them to hand over that control. Being aware of this, can be helpful while familiarizing yourself with the state of their financial affairs.

2. Organizing documentation for parents. Locating your loved ones' legal documents is the first task in organizing their financial estate. There are key documents to search for including:

- Birth certificates
- Marriage certificates
- Social Security cards
- Life, health and property insurance policies
- Mortgage information
- Keys or combinations to safes or safety deposit boxes
- Account numbers and passwords to bank accounts
- Information about stocks, bonds, or retirement accounts

3. Organize Estate Planning Documents. Does your parent or loved one have the documents listed here?

- A living will
- A last will
- A living trust (also titled Health Care Directive)
- A power of attorney

These are necessary documents, so if they do not exist, it would be wise to find an attorney and have them drawn up. A last will and testament and a living will are both necessary for estate planning. If your loved one owns valuable property, they may also need a living trust, as this protects the monetary value of these assets from probate.

There are different types of powers of attorney. A durable power of attorney for finances only allows your loved one to choose someone to perform financial transactions for them, should they be mentally or physically unable to do so for themselves. It can be written to take effect only after a specific event happens. Some examples of such an event would be dementia, the death of a spouse, or an incapacitating sickness. The durable power of attorney will allow your loved one to maintain control of their finances for as long as possible.

A health care power of attorney is usually written up in combination with a living will. It outlines your loved ones' own individual health care desires in advance, so that when they become unable to make those decisions for themselves, they are assured that a trusted person is following through on their wishes. An example of this would be writing up a 'Do Not Resuscitate' order.

It is always wise to prepare for future problems in advance. So, give an attorney a call and ask for assistance in preparation. Doing so will help ease the additional burden of being the financial caretaker for your loved one.

There are a lot of resources to help you; specifically you can download the Go-to-Packet for Grandparents at http://caregiversadvisors.org/go-to, to help you organize important information. Always remember that you are not alone.

Chapter 4- Choosing Nursing Care for Your Loved One with Alzheimer's

There may come a time when you are no longer able to take care of your loved one on your own. Caring for a person with advanced Alzheimer's or dementia is a full time job, and can require a team to accomplish. Thankfully, there are many options available.

If you are able to keep your loved one with Alzheimer's or dementia at home, but need help with the daily care, in home nursing is certainly an option. There are many agencies that send home health aides, state tested nurse aides, licensed practical nurses, or registered nurses into your home. Each of these provides a different level of care for your loved one.

A home health aide often assists with daily living activities such as feeding, bathing, and entertaining your loved one. A state tested nurse aide may be able to do more medical tasks such as taking blood pressure and pulse, and both will record their activities and findings for the shift in a log. This will allow you to see how your loved one has been cared for while you are at work, even overnight while you are getting your rest. Home health aides and STNA's are available to stay for two to 12 hour shifts with your loved one. LPN's and RN's come for visits as needed to assess your loved one's condition, and prescribe or administer medications needed.

You may only need to find short term care for your loved one while you are going on vacation, or during a difficult time, such as when you or someone you are close to are undergoing surgery. Home health agencies may provide care, depending on the length of time needed. If out of home care is necessary, a nursing home is a good option. Finding the right facility can be a challenging chore, yet there are a variety of ways they can help.

Short term assisted living facilities can be utilized when your loved one is capable of being alone for short periods of time. They provide many valuable services. Cooking meals for your loved one, cleaning your loved one's living quarters, transporting them to a doctor's office or bringing medical services to the patient, safety checks, and encouragement of independence as possible.

If your loved one's disease has progressed to the point of needing full time supervision, long term care is most likely the route you will need to go. The goal of a long term facility is to care for your loved one as you would, while providing in house medical services. Some things to consider while searching for a long term care facility are:

- Accreditation by State agencies
- Recommendation by word of mouth
- Listed on sites such as Angie's List that give reviews by current consumers
- Staff to meet the needs of your loved one in line with your budgeting needs

Take your time while looking for a place to care for your loved one long term. Most likely this will be where they will be spending their last days. You want to be sure that the facility you choose is staffed with people who care greatly for the elderly and will do their best to keep your loved one as comfortable as possible.

Chapter 5- Is Home Health Care the Best Decision for My Loved One?

Home health care is unfortunately something that we all might have to consider one day. No one wants to think about the fact that we could someday have to care for our aging parents, Unfortunately with Alzheimer's and other health issues on the rise; we could one day be put in the position where we must make a choice between a nursing home facility and home health care.

A lot of people have chosen to go with home health care. If you are in a position to care for a parent in your home and you choose not to place them in a nursing home, there are a few things you need to know and do to give them the best care possible.

First consult with the doctor to make sure your loved one is able to be cared for at home, depending on the circumstances you may not have the proper knowledge, space in your home, or the right equipment, and training to give best care.

Make sure you know all the requirements to caring for the patient, such as what is their diagnosis, what medicines they are taking, when to administer the medications, what type of treatments they require, can you give the treatments yourself or will nursing assistance be required, and if so, how much it is going to cost on a monthly basis to have a nurse come in to administer the treatments.

Caring for a parent in your home is very rewarding and fulfilling, but also time consuming, so make sure you are able to adjust your life to accommodate this change, you do not want to realize to late that you cannot handle the situation. It is better to make the right decision from the start, otherwise it can be emotionally damaging to you and the one you are caring for.

If possible take a course in health care or at least make sure you do a lot of research. This will help you to better understand what you are supposed to be doing and what the proper way to take care of your loved one is. There are a lot of complex issues that can and will arise from caring for a parent in your home especially if memory loss is an issue or your loved one is disabled and cannot move around on their own. Make sure you know CPR, taking the basic exam can end saving the life of the person you are caring for.

Sometimes with the memory loss that comes with aging, it can be heartbreaking to see your parent forget who you are or how to do things they have always done. This can make it difficult to care for your parent or loved one. So make sure you know who to contact for help and support when or if the time comes that you need it.

It is a good idea to have someone who is qualified to be able to relieve you sometimes in your role as care giver. It can be emotionally and physically and tiring to constantly care for someone if you are on your own. The stress that builds up can cause you to become depressed, lose focus and possibly make mistakes that can lead to accidents.

It is highly recommended that you take time for yourself to relax and calm your mind so you will be able to give the best care to your parent or loved one. We all want to do what we feel is right for the ones that need our help, but what you need to decide is what is the best course of action that will give your loved one the proper care that they need. Making these decisions are, at best, tough, and at worst, heartbreaking. So make sure you have all the information before you proceed. This will save you any emotional turmoil that can arise from a wrong choice.

Chapter 6 - Helping Those Caring for Parents with Alzheimer's and Dementia

One of the biggest stressors on a family has to care for a sick loved one. This is increasingly so when the illness begins to affect the judgment and rational of the family member who has fallen ill. Families caring for parents with Alzheimer Disease and other forms of Dementia know all too well the struggles of caring for a loved one who can no longer care for themselves. Families who find they are struggling to care for their parents should seek the services of hospitals and health care facilities to teach them methods of not only to care for their parents, but also making their parents as comfortable as possible. Healthcare professionals are readily available to begin working with family on parental care to ensure that the process is as manageable as possible.

Expect Changes

The everyday dynamics in the home for the family and Alzheimer's or Dementia suffering parent will drastically change. This can have a profound effect on everyone involved. Medical and social work experts can help families prepare for the changing dynamics. And although the dynamics in the home are changing the parent who is ill will need an environment that is very familiar to them. This can be a difficult task to keep life as familiar to the parent as possible in spite of how much everyday life has changed. Although difficult, this is not an impossible task to accomplish with the assistance of the right professional help.

Enhance Understanding

Another important aspect that a healthcare professional can assist a family and Dementia or Alzheimer's suffering parent is helping the caregivers understand fully what their parent is going through. The family who is providing the care must understand in full detail the severity of what their parent is going through. This is so the family will not have unrealistic expectations of what their suffering parent could do or comprehend. This will alleviate a great amount of stress off of both the family and the suffering parent.

Coping Techniques

Coping techniques will be vital for both the caregivers and parent. The parent suffering from the illness will have to be guided through ways for them to cope with everyday life. This may be accomplished by doing things as simple as: labeling the refrigerator, light, bathroom, television, etc. This may also entail education on how to speak and communicate with the parent in order that it minimizes them feeling frightened or frustrated. Caregivers must also learn coping techniques for themselves. It will not be easy caring for a parent with Alzheimer's or other forms of Dementia. This can bring on a great deal of frustration on the part of the caregiver. Health care professionals and social workers can train caregivers in ways to avoid becoming stressed, or dealing with stress should it occur.

Because of the challenging tasks of caring for a parent with any form of Dementia, families should heavily consider seeking the service of health care professionals in order to ensure a stable and safe environment for all who are involved.

Chapter 7 - Working with Doctors and Memory Loss Patients

Switching roles from your parent's child to your parent's caregiver is a difficult road. There are so many avenues that you must consider. After learning about a lot of other physical concerns of the elderly patient, you will most likely need to tackle one of the most confusing to navigate, memory loss. This is an area that is not yet fully understood by doctors. It is also a reality that each patient will face individual concerns when dementia or Alzheimer's disease begins to take over.

Working with doctors on patients with memory loss is the best way to educate yourself. Find a doctor who is compassionate, knowledgeable, and willing to take the time to get to know your loved one. You can Google, "doctors and Alzheimer's" or "doctors and dementia" to find a health care provider. This will greatly benefit you, as your doctor will observe and work with your loved one on his or her particular issues. There isn't a simple, single test that can diagnose a person with Alzheimer's or dementia. The diagnosis is a process, made by a doctor when they have done a complete analysis and assessment of your loved ones' symptoms and the possible causes.

The process begins in the doctor's office during the medical workup. Your loved one's health care provider will look over his or her medical history. The provider will ask several questions. The questions will be directed towards your loved one, who is having memory issues. Helping your loved one to answer them is one of the reasons you, or someone else close to your loved one, who is aware of his or her symptoms should be present for this visit.

1. Please list your current and past illnesses.

2. Explain key medical conditions that other family members have had in the past or have currently, including Alzheimer's, dementia, or any significant signs of memory loss.

3. List the medications you are currently taking, including natural health supplements.

4. What are some of the problems you are experiencing?

5. When did you first observe them?

6. How often do you notice the symptoms?

7. Have the symptoms increased?

8. Please detail your nutritional intake, including the use of alcohol.

There will also be physical tests the health care provider will perform:

1. Blood pressure, temperature, and pulse will be taken.

2. The heart and lungs will be listened to and assessed.

3. Blood and urine samples will be obtained and tested in a laboratory.

The information obtained from the physical examination can help identify other health issues your loved one is experiencing that could cause or intensify their symptoms of dementia or Alzheimer's disease. They will help the health care provider determine if your loved one is truly entering the beginning stages of dementia or Alzheimer's. Other conditions that can mimic or cause the symptoms of memory loss and trouble focusing include:

- Anemia
- Heart Problems
- Depression
- Lung Problems
- Infection
- Certain vitamin deficiencies
- Liver disease
- Thyroid irregularities

Once the health care provider has ruled out the above issues, it may be easier for them to pinpoint the symptoms your loved one is experiencing as the beginning stages of dementia or Alzheimer's disease. Should this be the case, the doctor could provide you and your loved one with a list of resources that will give you a community, support, and help answering your questions.

Chapter 8 - Getting the Needed Support

Because Alzheimer's is a progressive and irreversible brain disease, once diagnosed, patients and their families must learn how to cope with what each new day brings. As they face issues like dementia, the patient is robbed of memory and learning ability. It is essential that families face the hurdles together, and Alzheimer's and dementia support groups become a source of daily strength and encouragement.

Support groups provide a myriad of services to patients and families. It is important for families to connect to resources that allow them to find competent caregivers. These give them not only important medical services, but they also allow breaks for those who stay with patients full time. This is also a safe place to share, exchange information, talk through concerns, and talk about coping and challenges that they face each day. These groups have trained leaders, experienced in this area.

One such group is The Alzheimer's Association. This nation-wide service can be found at www.alz.org, and it is a valuable resource for so many suffering. Founded in 1980, this organization "advances research to end Alzheimer's and dementia, while enhancing care for those living with the disease." Patients and families have access to 24/7 Helpline, and there are local chapters all across the United States. With more than 5 million Americans suffering from this disease, many people seek this help on a daily basis. By typing in a zip code or area, it is easy to find local help near anyone.

If patients prefer internet support groups, ALZConnected is a complete source of online help. Here patients and families can access a myriad of message boards, seeking out others to ask questions or just voice concerns. There are lists of community activities and solutions for many issues that arise. Many people come here to just share struggles, and those who respond, understand. The quote that seems to sum up this site is posted: "At ALZConnected, I don't have to explain what it means to live with Alzheimer's." This is a common sentiment, as this difficult disease often brings many questions, anguish, and pain, and when others can share their own stories, they are comforted to know that someone else has gone through the same.

The message boards also provide specialized help for several different groups affected by this disease. There is a Caregiver Forum, designed to help those who are constantly caring for these patients. A Spouse or Partner Caregiver Forum also meets the needs of those whose lives change, as their lifetime partner suddenly struggles to do what they used to do. Finally another forum is for Younger Onset Dementia. This deals with the unique issues facing young children and their families.

ALZConnected also has a specific area specifically for Solutions. This allows anyone to ask any question, and they will get a solution to this inquiry in the form of many, many caring individuals who seek to make other's lives easier. Often they have gone through the same issues, and this is what will give them that peace of mind to deal with difficult moments in life. Often times, questions are greeted with a large number of responses. Those who deal with this disease are eager to help others.

Other support groups are also available in many communities. It is quite simple to find such sources online; some examples include Area Agency on Aging and Alzheimer's Family Services. These groups are most often free, and they offer complete privacy and respect for all patients, family members, and caregivers.

Coping with Alzheimer's and the dementia that comes from this disease, can be one of the most painful experiences a family can go through. As the patient slowly loses daily functions and ability to recognize and remember, it is crucial to find support. With the care and love provided by Alzheimer's and dementia support groups, families are able to cope, and the patient is able to live life with dignity.

Chapter 9- Communication with an Alzheimer's Patient

Communication can be difficult with anyone at times. Keeping in mind what type of emotional state the other person is in is always a good idea. When a person feels confused or frustrated they are likely to act out. People who are suffering from dementia or Alzheimer's disease can feel confused and frustrated most of the time, making communication difficult.

When your parent is the one suffering from one of these diseases, it can be doubly difficult. Your parents have always taken care of you, and it can feel overwhelming to have become your parents' caregiver. Learning how to communicate with parents with Alzheimer's or dementia is necessary to help smooth the transition from the role of child to the role of caregiver.

Listening skills, understanding, patience, and a feel for emotional vibes are all required to communicate well with an Alzheimer's or dementia patient. The information and techniques below will be helpful, assisting you in salvaging much of your relationship with your ailing parent.

Communication Changes

In the early stages of Alzheimer's or dementia, your parents' communication may well remain basically unchanged. As their disease progresses you may begin to see more noticeable changes.

- More Silent Times – your parent may being to have more time periods in which they just don't talk

- Disorganized Speaking – They may begin speaking, only to stop and start again because the words are not coming out in the order that they wanted them to.

- Switching Languages - If your parent has a native language, he or she may begin speaking it rather than the secondary language they have spoken for so long.

- Forgetting What They Were Saying – They may lose track of what they were just talking about.

- New Words – Your parent may not remember what familiar items are called, and may make up random new words to describe them

- Repetition – Your parent may repeat words over and over

Helping Your Parent Communicate

- Patience and Support – These cannot be over stated. Listen, wait, and watch until you are sure you know what your parent is attempting to communicate.

- Avoid being demanding or critical – This will not help them, in fact it may cause them to physically act out and accidentally hurt themselves.

- Offer Alternatives – Offer your parent a comb, a washcloth, a different shirt, whatever it is that you think that they may need.

- Offer Comfort – When they are appearing to get frustrated, hold their hand, or pat it, making sure that they know that you care about what they are trying to communicate.

- Avoid arguing – Even if your parent says something that does not make sense, avoid trying to correct them. This will only aggravate communication.

- Pay Attention to Feelings Instead of Words – This is where the emotional vibes come in. Knowing that your parent's overall feeling of frustration trumps what exactly he or she is saying, try to be compassionate. They will know what you are feeling.

Tips and Tricks for Late Stage Dementia or Alzheimer's

Later in the disease' progression, wording will matter less, body language and tone will matter more.

- Stay calm – As we discussed earlier, these diseases are confusing and frustrating for the patient. The less aggravation, the better.

- Keep Your Sentences Short and Simple – the less there is to get confused about, the better off your communication will be.
- Speak slowly and distinctively – Again, use the least amount of confusion possible

- Repeat Information As Needed

- Answer Questions, rather than ask them– For example say, "The bathroom is this way." Instead of asking, "Do you have to go to the bathroom?"

Communication at any age can be difficult. Follow these tips, and you should experience greater results!

Chapter 10 - Helping Kids Understand Alzheimer's and Dementia

You have come so far in understanding the disease that your parent or loved one is going through. Now you need to help the children in your loved one's life understand. Helping kids understand dementia can be difficult. Depending on the age of the child, they may or may not possess the mental capabilities to process such a situation. Assuming that the patient with the disease is a grandparent, it may be hard for the child to understand why grandma or grandpa has changed so much.

There are multiple factors that will determine how much or how little the child will be affected.

1. How closely the child is related to the person with the disease.

2. How close the child or teen is to the patient emotionally.

3. How close in physical proximity the patient is to the child or teen. Have they always lived hours apart? Or does their loved one live next door?

The ways in which the child will be affected vary as well. When their loved one is suffering from dementia or Alzheimer's they may react in one or many of these ways:

1. They may feel sadness.

2. They may be curious about what is causing this.

3. May feel confused. Why is their loved one acting this way?

4. They may be frustrated by the new ways they must interact with their loved one, such as having to repeat themselves multiple times.

5. Teen or older child may feel guilty for resenting the time and effort spent on caring for their loved one.

6. They may experience fear of their loved ones new actions, or of what will happen to their loved one in the future.

7. They may worry that they will get the disease.

8. They may be embarrassed to bring their friends around the patient because of their loved ones' strange actions.

9. They may be unsure of what to do or how to act around this "new" person that used to be so different.

It is normal for the child to feel all of these things. Kids bounce back relatively easily, and will most likely respond to the situation better than most adults. Encourage the child to write down their feelings in a journal. Journaling can be comforting.

Helping kids understand dementia or other related diseases are a case in which honesty is the best policy. It is important not to lie to them. Acknowledge the reality that grandma or grandpa will not be getting better, and that the best course of action is to enjoy the time that we have with them.

It may also help to share the details of the disease, how it will progress, and what changes will be made to accommodate grandma or grandpa. Talking to kids on their level will help them get a grasp on the situation. Use words that they understand, like "grandma forgets things sometimes, and she will begin to forget more often". Children will probably notice their loved one getting progressively worse, so it only makes sense to clue them in ahead of time.

Giving the child positive ways to interact with their loved one will be another great tool in helping them deal with the situation. Encourage them to play games with grandma or grandpa. Watch movies with them, and listen to songs that their loved one enjoys. Breaking the news and helping them understand may be difficult at first, but you may be surprised at the compassion children can display, and how well they can deal with their loved one's disease.

Chapter 11 - Elderly Exercises

Doing exercises with the elderly may be a challenge but, it will be well worth it. The expression "Use it or lose it" in many cases can be true. It is more important foe muscles to be toned and to have strong bones now than when you were young. When you live a sedentary life as an elderly person it can cause you not to be able to get in certain positions, to bend over, squat, walk, stay balanced and the ability to be flexible.

But, seniors shouldn't be expected to do exercises they didn't even do when they were younger, like skiing or playing tennis. This could be dangerous and the body might have a hard time making the adjustment to anything strenuous. Due to muscle weakness and balance sometimes it is a miracle for them just to be able to move around or walk on their own without falling.

However, with this being said, it is important for an elderly person to have a physical activity worked into their daily routine. As we age so do our internal organs, and the joints and spine start to degenerate and the muscle fibers shorten. So as we get older we need to continue to exercise to improve our strength, flexibility, balance, and to improve blood circulation.

Working the muscles everyday is very important and most of the exercises for the elderly are done with the help of a chair. This gives them security and balance as they start their exercises. This consists of slow movements and stretches that are held working the upper part of the body while using the chair to sit in. To maintain their balance using the chair they work their legs and lower back with bends and flexes. When they do this muscle building exercises and toning exercises, they gain more strength, balance and flexibility. As this happens, to build up the muscles even more, they will be able to add a little weight for toning to their daily activity. Even a daily walk is great exercise.

If the elderly have access to a swimming pool it is one of the best options for physical activity as it helps them build and tone their muscle. Using the resistance of the water as they move their bodies through it creates a muscle toning session that can be beneficial to them as well as enjoyable. Even a daily walk is great exercise. Start some of these exercises at home with the family. Have some family exercise routines together; it can be beneficial as well as fun. If nothing else, maybe walk together.

Listed below are some of the elderly exercise routines that can be offered:

- The Seated Core Stretch
- The Standing Twist
- Stand up toe reach
- Double arm reach and leg lift
- Calf exercise routine
- Neck rotation exercise
- Shoulder lateral exercise
- Back exercise routine
- If you are in decent shape and want to do more there are plenty of videos that offer exercises along with dancing to the elderly.

As you move through your life and your body starts to slow down also remember that body exercises are important, but also your mind exercises as extremely important. Do something to keep your brain alive, functioning and very active. Listed below are some clues of what to do:

- Reading
- Game of memory
- SUDOKU
- Playing a string instrument like the guitar
- Painting (art)
- Puzzles
- Transcendental Meditation
- Video and computer games
- Active learning

Chapter 12 - Tips for Caregivers of Alzheimer's Patients

When you are caring for an elderly person with Alzheimer's disease, there is a lot to remember. While you are trying to keep all the information you are learning regarding your loved one's care, you are also juggling the physical demands of their care. People with Alzheimer's in its early stages can still be physically active and unpredictable in their actions. You may feel as though you are caring for an adult sized child, and this is not very far from the truth. Caring for a person with Alzheimer's is a labor of love. To help make this a little simpler, let's go over some helpful tips.

Personal Care and Hygiene

People who suffer from Alzheimer's can become quite agitated when you attempt to dress or undress them, bathe them, apply deodorant or brush their teeth. There are a few things to remember during these times.

- No sudden movements– Alzheimer's sufferers feel more secure when you move slowly.

- Always tell them what you are about to do– Don't take them off guard

- Don't be forceful or demanding- too often caregivers get frustrated that when a patient or loved one refuses to brush their teeth or comb their hair. The best method is to employ a calm demeanor and ask nicely.

- Exercise patience– when your loved one refuses treatment, just remember that it is the nature of their disease to forget quickly. When they refuse to brush their teeth, just smile, nod, and try again a few minutes later. Odds are they will be much more agreeable.

Medications

This part of the care giving process is probably one of the most simple to organize. Once you have gotten the right types of medications there are really only three things to know.

- Use a daily or weekly pill organizer – these little inventions are life savers and pretty self explanatory.

- Keep medication bottles and organizers in a safe hiding place.

- Individuals with Alzheimer's will eat a lot of things, just as a child would.

- Be sure to give medications on time.

Home care Activities

It is amazing how much time it takes to care for an individual with Alzheimer's. It is probably comparable to bringing home a new baby. Keep your loved one fed, bathed, and properly rested and medicated will take up much of your day. There may be some time in between these personal care routines that could be spent just enjoying the time you have with your loved one. Even if your loved one has progressed in their disease to the point of not being fully aware or comprehensive, these activities may still interest them.

- Putting together a puzzle
- Watching a favorite TV show
- Playing Cards
- Reading a Book
- Folding wash cloths or Napkins

Outings with Alzheimer's Patients

Doctor's appointments and grocery store runs are two of the most common reasons for leaving the house with your loved one. A few tips to remember on these outings are:

• Take your patience with you – this cannot be overstated.

• Alzheimer's patients can be difficult to manage in a home setting, not to mention a public place.

• Take entertainment to the doctor's office. A book or magazine may be just the thing to help your loved one make it through the waiting period.

• Bring extra clothing – elderly people are sensitive to changes in temperature. It may be sweltering outside, yet freezing in the doctor's office due to air conditioning.

- Bring a list of medications if going to the doctor's office. He or she will need to know what your loved one is already taking before prescribing anything new.

- Take a grocery list if your outing is for groceries. There's no worse fate than forgetting that once necessary ingredient for tonight's supper, and when you are out with an Alzheimer's patient things can get exciting fast and cause you to forget.

Employing these tips should help make your care giving days run a little more smoothly. Don't forget to take time off for yourself as well!

Chapter 13- When Caring for an Alzheimer's Patient

Caring for patients suffering from Alzheimer's disease can be difficult. As the condition progresses, patients begin to show a significant increase in some symptoms such as: impaired thinking, severe memory loss, confusion, relentlessness, impaired judgment, language deterioration and the inability to follow simple directions. When medical staff diligently follows hospital procedures during times when Alzheimer patients are not having a good day, they will be able to give these patients the type of care needed to get them through rough times. It is important for staff to know the everyday methods of making patients comfortable; as well as knowing what to do in an emergency to ensure the safety and well-being of the patient.

Speaking With Families

As families begin to inquire about hospitalizing Alzheimer patients it is important for medical staff to assure that the family is well informed of all that will take place during the process. Hospital staff should explain to families the emergency procedures that are used to ensure safety, the various techniques used to help patients experience as less discomfort as possible, and exercises used to help the patients stay become easier.

Helping Patients Cope with Every Day Life

There are various methods that can be used to help patients have as less frustration and discomfort in their everyday life. For instance: being that these patients will be suffering from memory loss, use large cards to label certain items in their room. Also, hospital staff should maintain a quiet environment for the patient. Loud noises can scare a patient and place them in a bad panic situation. If there is to be a television or radio in the room, be sure that both are always kept at a moderate volume.

Communicating with Alzheimer Patients

Hospital staff should always remember to introduce themselves in a calm and tender demeanor. New faces can be a frightening experience for patients. Staff should also speak slowly so the patient can process what the staff is saying. Good eye contact is important. Approaching a patient from behind is never a good idea. Staff should always be sure to display a calm loving demeanor toward the patient. Nonverbal communication can also be utilized once the patient begins to become comfortable with the staff. A gentle touch in these situations is a good idea when appropriate.

What to Do In an Emergency?

In cases of emergencies Alzheimer patients should NEVER be left alone. As hospital staff is trying to calm the situation, they cannot show any signs of fret or over anxiousness. Make sure that questions are made simple for the patients. Usually yes or no questions work best- as they do not force too much thinking on the patient during a time they are disorientated. Hospital staff must keep close eye contact when speaking to a patient in these situations. Staff must be mindful of what they say in front of the patient. Although there may be a crisis the patient is experiencing, they can still hear. And the wrong words said can make the situation extremely worse.

Following proper hospital procedure while caring for an Alzheimer patient can go a long way with the patient being as comfortable and safe as possible during their stay.

Chapter 14- Understanding Memory Loss

Alzheimer's disease will usually come in a seven step process, but all the symptoms for AD will always vary from person to person, and so does the rate at which they change from stage to stage. This list of stages is only a general guideline of what the ability may be of someone, and how their abilities will change through the stages. These seven stages are based off a system designed by Barry Reisberg M.D.1.

Stage One – No loss or regular function. A patient in this stage does not have any problems remembering things, and will not show any symptoms as to any memory loss.

Stage Two – Very slight mental weakening. This stage can easily be confused with changes that are associated with age. A person in this stage may complain of having minor memory gaps such as forgetting where common objects are located, although they will not show any signs of dementia in a medical inspection.

Stage Three – Minor decline in mental strength. Signs of people in this stage include; difficulty remembering any newly introduced people, losing cherished objects, or seeing visible difficulty in them trying to perform daily tasks. During this stage, it is possible that the early parts of Alzheimer's can be diagnosed.

Stage Four – Temperate decline in mental health. In this point of the process, most medical practitioners should be able to diagnose with confidence. Someone in stage four will forget very current events, have trouble with most intellectual math, and forget about their own history.

Stage Five – reasonably serious decline in mental strength. During this stage, major breaks in the memory are very obvious, and they will need extra help with all their daily events. During this process people with Alzheimer's will be incapable of remembering any numbers such as the phone number or their address or they may not know where they are at, or even the day that it is.

Stage Six – Serious decline in mental strength. Someone is this stage will have memory that will continue to get worse and worse. They may also experience personality changes, and they will need a lot of assistance in day-to-day events. They may also need help getting dressed, or they may have a habit of running off, and getting lost.

Stage Seven – Very Serious decline in mental health: this is the very final stage of the disease. Someone in this stage may be incapable of continuing conversations, or movement. When they reach this point in the stage, the individuals will need extensive help with activities such as using the bathroom, eating, and any other daily activities. Again the stages are different for everyone, and most of the stages will overlap, so it is hard to put someone in one specific stage.

The stages of dementia are very similar to that of Alzheimer's, but they are in fact two different things. Dementia is a symptom, while Alzheimer's disease is a result of the symptom. Although, even though they are different, they have similar characteristics. Both of them are not reversible, and will generally come from aging.

Chapter 15 - Elderly Health Concerns

Family can be a wonderful thing. Your parents and your grandparents have always been there for you. As they age, they become less able to care for themselves. Now it's time for you to give them some return on their lifetime investment in your care. This time in your life can be a challenge. While you may still have children of your own at home, you are also learning about the health concerns of the elderly in order to care for that special person who has always taken care of you. You may be learning about elderly dental problems.

You may have had to take your relative to an elderly vision specialist for an exam. You may also have grown familiar with your loved ones' audiologist. Elderly hearing loss is probably one of the most common health issues that happen as we age. Because elderly health concerns may be a new area you are dealing with, let's go over three of the most common concerns. Here they are, from the diagnosis to the treatment options.

Gingivitis

Gingivitis is an infection of the gums that can lead to tooth loss if left untreated. Some symptoms include red, swollen or tender gums, gums that bleed, loose teeth, pain with chewing, or dentures that no longer fit. A diagnosis of gingivitis is made during a dental exam. The dentist may use a ruler to measure pockets around the teeth, or take an x-ray to look for bone loss. Gingivitis is an elderly health concern that is treatable. You may need to help your loved one practice proper oral hygiene, and ask them to cut back on smoking, as this will only slow the healing.

Glaucoma

It is estimated that nearly one million people in America over the age of 65 have some loss of vision due to glaucoma. Glaucoma is a buildup of fluid in the eye. This disease can be asymptomatic in its earlier stages. Symptoms that develop can include visual field loss, and as the disease progresses, blurred vision.

The diagnosis is made when the ophthalmologist discovers a rise in the normally low intraocular pressure, and then examines the optic nerve for damage. The first method of treatment for glaucoma is an eye drop that will increase the outflow or reduce the fluid buildup. More severe cases may require laser surgery. If caught early, glaucoma can be controlled, however if your loved one has waited too long, the damage cannot be undone.

Presbycusis

Presbycusis is hearing loss that is associated with old age. Changes occur in the auditory nerve, middle, inner, and outer ears that cause this condition. Hearing tests are done at the audiologist's office to determine the extent of the damage. Hearing aids that go into the ear, as well as other aids such as higher volume appliances or even wireless headphones can be purchased for speaking on the phone, or watching television.

How your loved one responds to any of the above mentioned diagnoses will be in part up to them, and in part up to you. They may find the changes difficult to understand. You may need to help them understand, as well as develop some coping mechanisms. Coping mechanisms can be both emotional and physical. Emotional coping mechanisms include techniques like "taking each day as it comes", and "looking on the bright side."

Physical coping mechanisms can be using a hearing aid, or remembering to floss. How you approach the situation is key. Keep an upbeat disposition and treat your time together as a life adventure. More than likely, you will have fun, learn a lot, and your elderly loved one will be very grateful for all that you do for them.

Recommended Reading

In researching for my own family, I found these to be helpful. You can check them out on my site here:

http://CaregiversAdvisors.org/Recommended

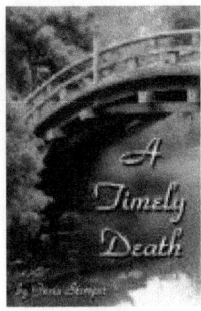

A Timely Death

A book that explores the meaningful relationship of a family, the damage that Alzheimer's brought, and the lengths that we are willing to reach for the ones we love.

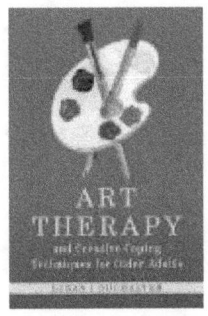

Art Therapy and Creative Coping Techniques for Older Adults

Suitable for older adults, including those with anxiety, depression or in the early stages of dementia, this will be an essential tool for art therapists as well as counsellors, carers, psychotherapists, and social workers.

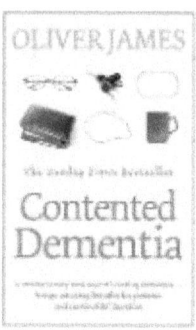

Contented Dementia: 24-hour Wraparound Care for Lifelong Well-being

A Dementia patient will usually experience random and frequently increased memory blanks to recent events. However, their feelings remain the same and the memories of past events are intact. Both of these can be utilize in a special way to replace for the recent information that has been lost. The SPECAL method (Specialized Early Care for Alzheimer's) outlined in this book works by creating links between past memories and the routine activities of daily life in the present.

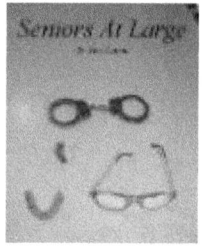

Seniors At Large

Eight elderly patients escaped their nursing home due to mistreatment. They had a hilarious, fun filled adventure, before ultimately redeeming themselves.

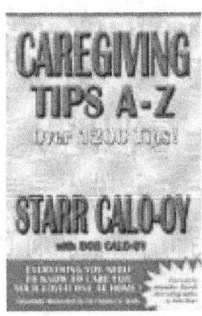

Caregiving Tips A-Z

All you need to know in providing care for your loved ones at home!

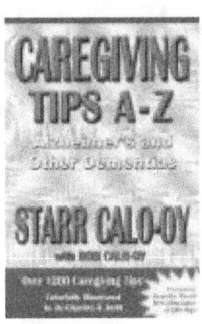

Caregiving Tips A-Z Alzheimer's & Other Dementias

All you need to know in providing care for your loved ones at home, especially the ones with Alzheimer's and Dementia.

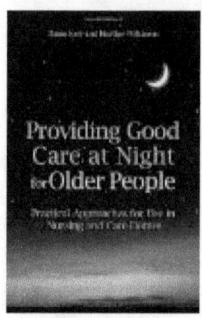

Providing Good Care at Night for Older People: Practical Approaches for Use in Nursing and Care Homes

This should be a good reference for night staff and their managers and employers, as well as inspectors of services, policy makers, and anyone else with an interest in the provision of care for older people.

About The Author

Doctor Jack Rosenberg – Board Certified physician. Graduated high school in Phoenix, Arizona as a member of the class of 1981. He later attended college where he received his B.S, Bachelors of Science degree, in Biology at the University of Arizona. There he graduated with Suma Cum Laude, High Distinction and Honors as a 1986 graduate. He was also a member of the Phi Beta Kappa. A strong advocate for excellence and education, he involved himself with continuing education and hard work. Doctor Rosenberg attended Medical school at the Medical College of Wisconsin (Marquette University) and graduated in 1991. For his residency he worked at the William Beaumont Hospital in Royal Oak, Michigan specializing in Obstetrics and Gynecology finishing in 1995. His professional interests focus on the health of others, helping others, and hard work to better others which lead to him creating his own private practice in Prescott, Arizona since 1997.

Doctor Rosenberg has garnered many high achievements that have helped others in his community as well as better himself. Education is of high importance to him as proven through his hard work and dedication to his goals and choices in life. He has made himself as well as his family proud. He is a true leader to his community. He likes hiking, tennis, boating, and spending time with his family. In addition, he serves as the husband of his beautiful wife of 23 years Jennifer Rosenberg. He also serves as the father of two children Collin and Beverly. Jennifer's mother has dementia and has been living with the Rosenberg's for about a year. Dementia is a brain disorder that cause memory disorders such as Alzheimer's. Doctor and Mrs. Rosenberg dedicate their time, not only to their careers, but also to their family and friends. Doctor Jack Rosenberg is of great excellence promoting education, family, aid, and more.

You can find Dr. Rosenberg on Google+ and Facebook. It is his purpose to empower caregivers of aging relatives to make good decisions for their loved ones health.

www.ingramcontent.com/pod-product-compliance
Lightning Source LLC
Chambersburg PA
CBHW071818170526
45167CB00003B/1356